The Little Book of
Loss & Grief

You can read while you
Cry

*This book is dedicated to my sister Mary Majella Crowe,
7 October 1969 – 2 August 1971, my first teacher in grief.*

*Also to the many precious children and families I have worked
with during my career who continue to teach me every day.
And to my own family with love.*

This book is a companion for anyone who has known the sadness of loss and grief.

Loss and grief are not just about death.

This book is for anyone who has ever suffered any kind of loss: divorce, infertility, unemployment, the end of a relationship, death, mental and physical health issues, conflict with loved ones, rejection – the list is endless.

This book is pretty much for us all.

This book will remind you that you are not alone.

That grief is normal.

That you are normal.

Grief can be a very lonely and frightening experience.

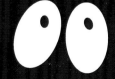

Grief can make you feel that everything you knew about the world has changed.

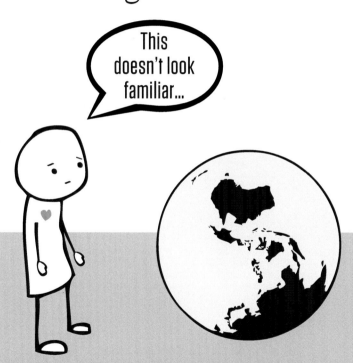

$\mathcal{A}$fter a loss you may feel like you are wearing a pair of invisible glasses.

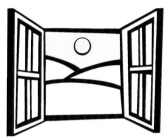

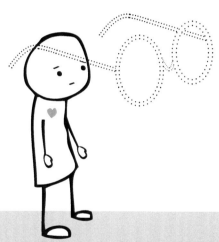

These glasses may give you a different view on life.
Your priorities may change ... or stay the same.
Whatever works for you is okay!

During Grief it can be hard to recognise yourself.

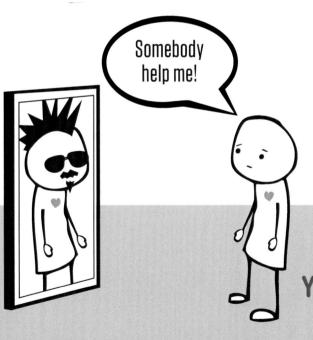

"What's happening to me?"
"Am I going crazy?"
"How did I become like this?"

You may worry that you will never feel 'normal' again.

It is still You in there!

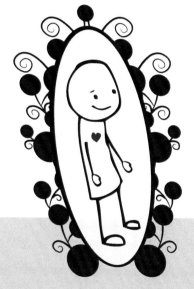 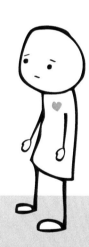

**It may be a *new* and *normal* you …
for a very *new* and *abnormal* situation.**

Grief is a very personal experience.
You can't compare your Grief to another person's Grief.

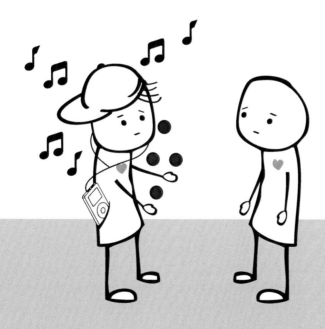

"I don't understand
what you are doing ..."

Your Grief may be hard for others to see or understand.

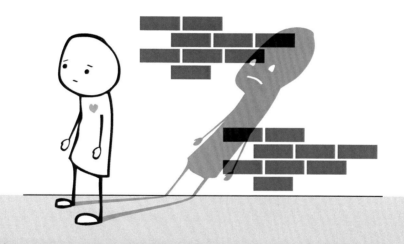

A bit like an unwanted dark shadow following you around.

Grief does not happen in stages or timeframes.

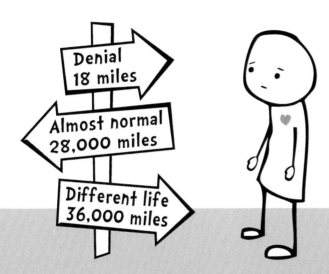

Denial
18 miles

Almost normal
28,000 miles

Different life
36,000 miles

Every person will have to find
their own way.

Grief cannot be measured.

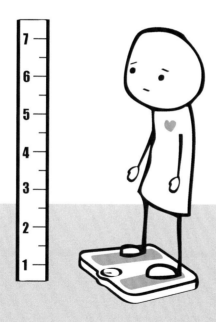

Grief cannot be weighed.

$\mathcal{G}$rief can be **exhausting**...

it can feel like a full-time job and may take all your energy.

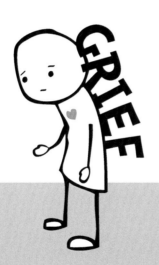

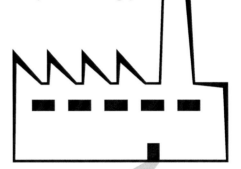

Be gentle with yourself.

Look after yourself.

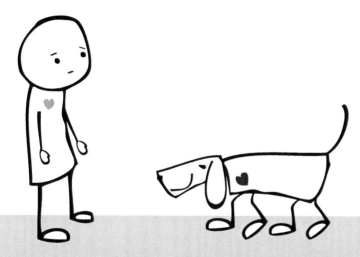

**Try to eat well, drink enough water and do some exercise.
Even very gentle walking may help lift the 'darkness'.
There are no big expectations. Start small.**

In times of loss, people may not know what to say or do.
This does not mean they do not care.

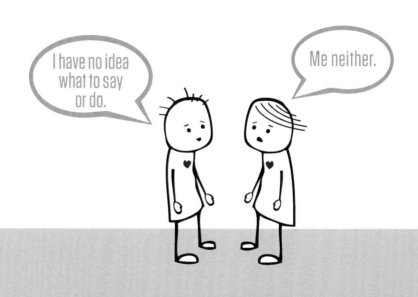

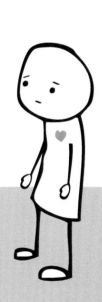

Find people who understand what you need to do for yourself.

Many people tie their Grief to guilt.

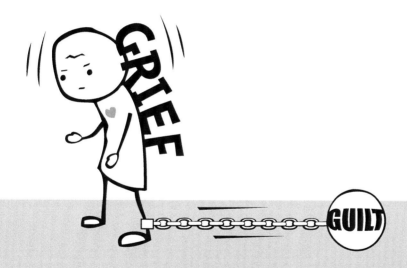

Guilt may be a very real part of grief – even though it is *rarely* anyone's fault.

Try not to invest too much time into guilt.
It won't change anything.

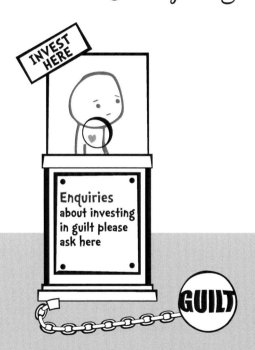

INVEST HERE

Enquiries about investing in guilt please ask here

GUILT

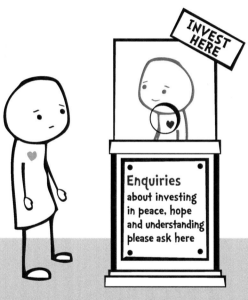

INVEST HERE

Enquiries about investing in peace, hope and understanding please ask here

Invest more time and energy into emotions that are helpful.

Sometimes you may need to take a break from your Grief.

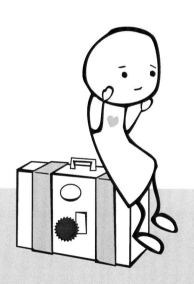

Destination:
Time out from Grief,
not staying long so
please enjoy your stay

It is still okay to laugh ...
to want to stop feeling so sad.

Your grief will probably still be there waiting for you when you get back.

Sometimes you may have to fight your way back from Grief.

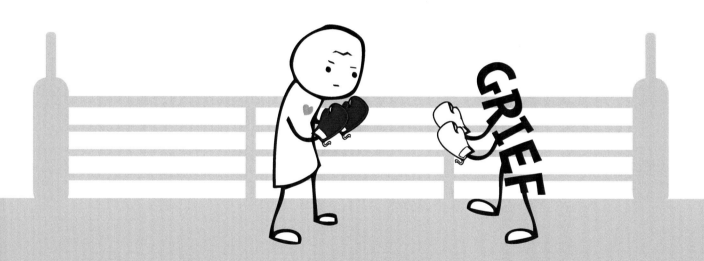

It may not just *'happen'*.

There is no such thing as 'normal' Grief.

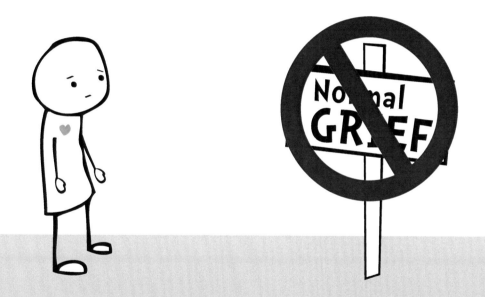

As long as you are not at risk of hurting yourself or others, what you are doing is normal for you.

The Myths of Crying.

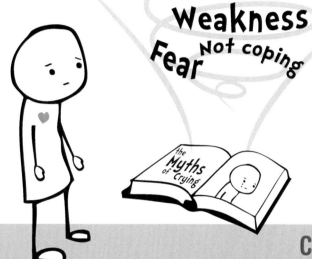

Weakness
Fear Not coping

Crying is not weakness.
Crying does not mean you are 'not coping'.
Crying is biological ... similar to a safety valve.
Try not to fear tears even if they are new to you.

Grief is not just about tears and crying.

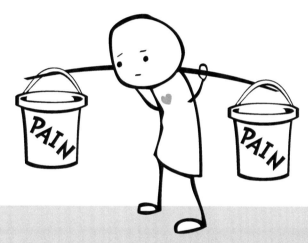

Some of us may cry _buckets_ of tears!
Some people may never cry a single tear but
still feel the heavy pain of grief.

Sometimes your tears will carry you to the next phase.

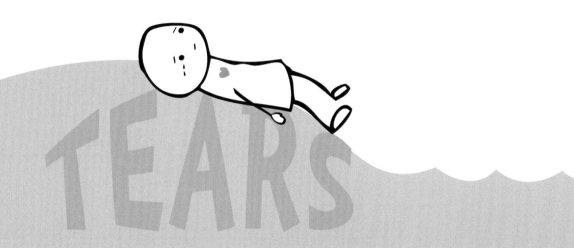

The way you grieve will depend on who you are and what has already happened in your life.

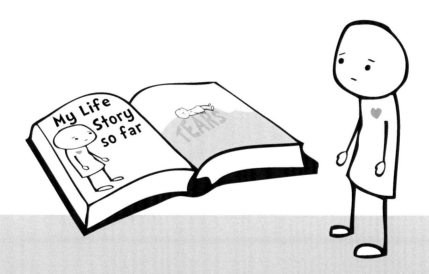

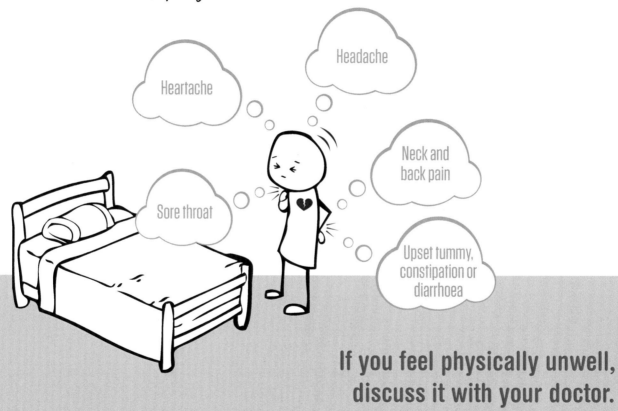

Grief can fill you with an **ANGER** and **RAGE** you have never known.

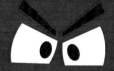

Other ways you may grieve (though this list is endless)...

You may eat too much,
or too little.

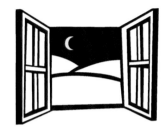

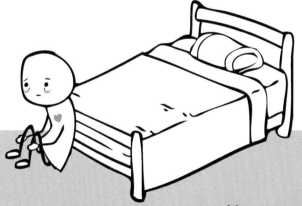

You may not be able to sleep.
You may find it hard to wake up and get going.

Using drugs or alcohol to numb the pain might seem like a good idea.

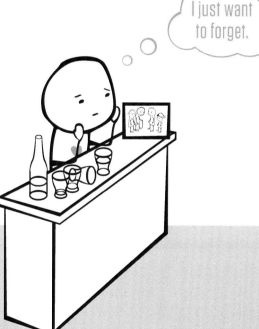

It never is.
Keep loved ones close.

When you are grieving you may come up with **big plans** or ideas simply because you want to be **distracted** from the pain.

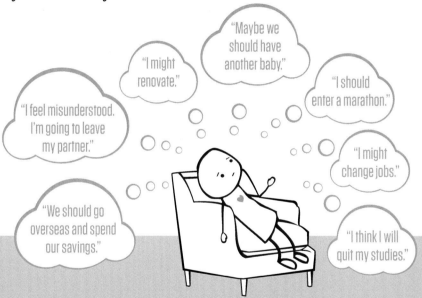

Move gently. Take your time before making any big life choices. Things may change again in the next days or weeks.

Your age may affect how you grieve.

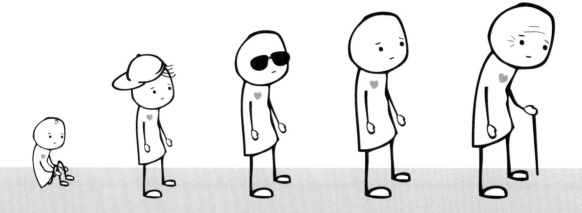

Age makes us understand the world in different ways.

Are you normally loud and chatty?

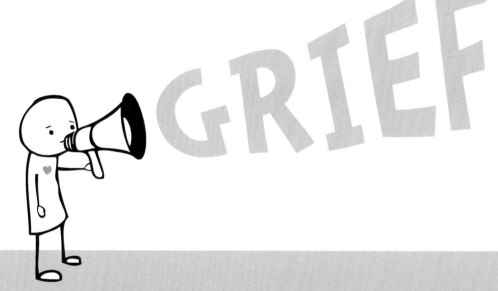

GRIEF

Sharing your story does not mean you are enjoying your Grief. You get energy from other people. It's how you cope.

Are you normally quiet and private?

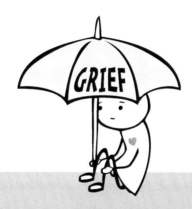

If you are a private person, keeping your Grief quiet may help you maintain your energy and survive.

In Grief there may be
times when you really want
to share and be with others.

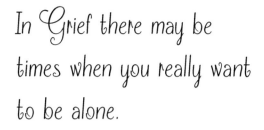

In Grief there may be
times when you really want
to be alone.

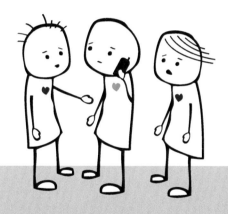

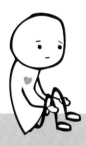

**This can change minute to minute
and that's okay.**

Grief can be expressed in many ways...

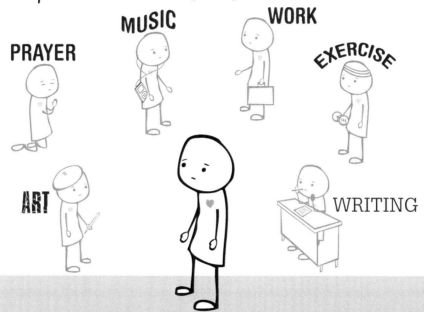

PRAYER

MUSIC

WORK

EXERCISE

ART

WRITING

It can be expressed energetically, through movement, exercise or dance. It can be expressed quietly, through meditation, stillness or mindfulness.

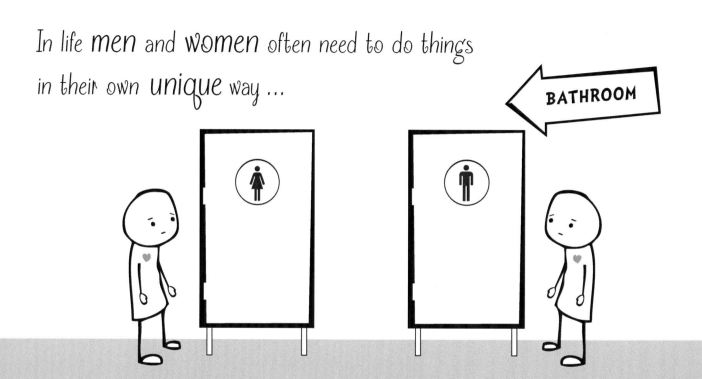

In Grief we are all going to have our own needs.

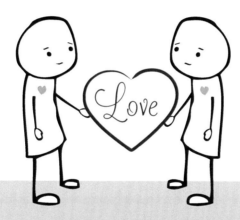

This will be true even in a relationship. If your Grief is shared, find ways to support and respect your partner even if what they are doing is not familiar to you.

$\mathcal{A}$ lot of what you have **learnt** over the years about $\mathcal{G}$rief comes from your **own** family.

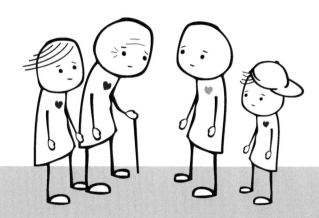

Keep this in mind, particularly if you are in a relationship.

Everyone thinks that the way **THEY** grieve is the right way.

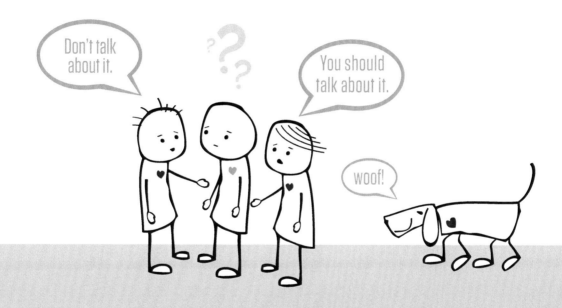

This can be hard if you are grieving with others.
There is no one **RIGHT** way to grieve.

Sometimes in Grief it can feel as if you have
fallen into a big, dark hole.

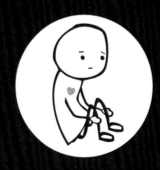

If you are in a hole and feel **frightened,**
call out to someone.

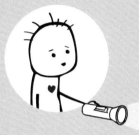

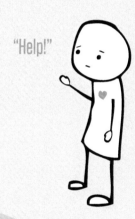

"Help!"

They may not be able to pull you out ...
but a friend or counsellor can always stand at the top and
shine a light to remind you that you are not alone.

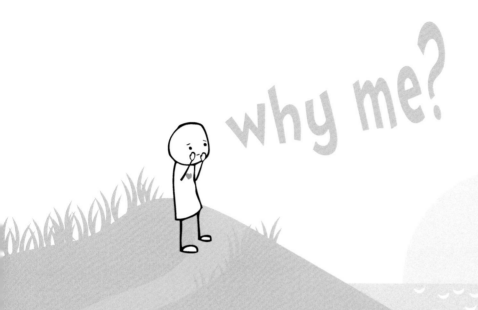

why me?

There is no justice or logic to loss.
Sometimes awful things just happen to wonderful people.

In Grief you may replay things over and over again in your head.

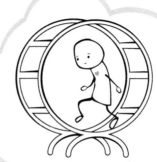

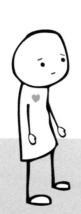

Try to create some quiet space.

Does time heal?

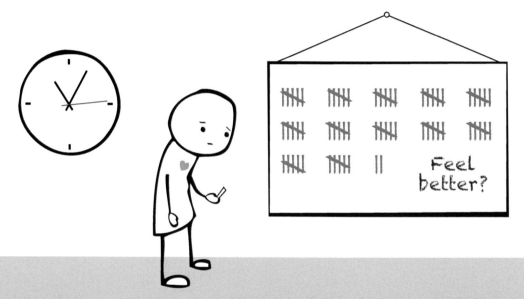

Feel better?

There is no magic timeframe for Grief,
though it may not always be as raw and painful as
it is in the early days, weeks, months or years.

Grief often leaves a scar... but that scar may not always ache as badly as it does today.

Ow that hurts!

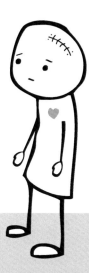

Grief can be unpredictable.
It can change day to day without warning.

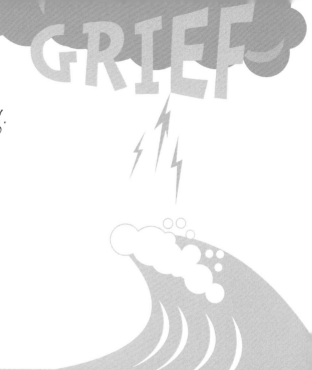

GRIEF

Ahh! Peace at last.

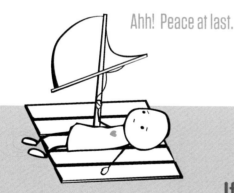

If grief returns wild and violent, remember that you have survived these days before.

There is no easy way to grieve.

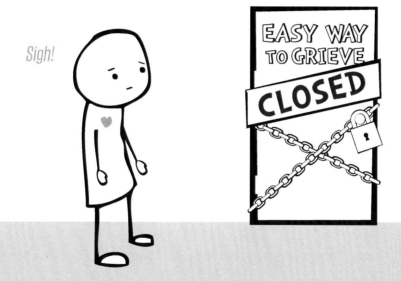

Everyone has their own story of Grief to tell.

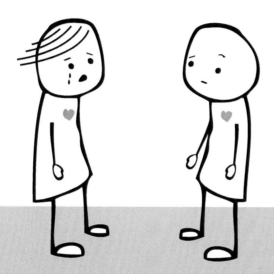

If you ask around you may be surprised what
others have survived before you.

Move very gently through this time.
Have no expectations or judgements of yourself.

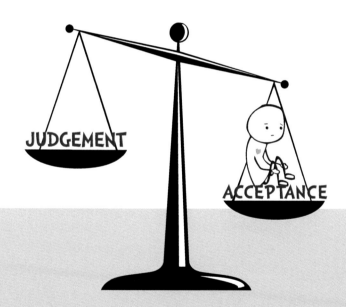

Find your own way in your own time.

Remember...

You are important.

Believe in the potential for things to change.

Grief is normal.

You are normal.

You are stronger than you think.

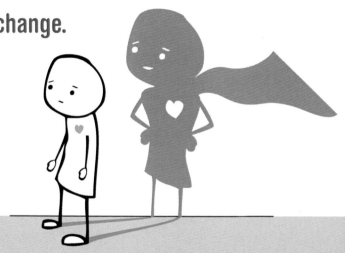

Be gentle with yourself.
Take care.

First published in 2014 by Liz Crowe

© Liz Crowe 2014

The moral rights of the author have been asserted

National Library of Australia Cataloguing-in-Publication entry:

Author:	Crowe, Liz, author.
Title:	The little book of loss & grief: you can read while you cry / Liz Crowe; Peter Reardon, illustrator.
ISBN:	9780992454104 (paperback)
Subjects:	Grief – Popular works.
	Loss (Psychology) – Popular works.
	Emotions – Popular works.
Other Authors/Contributors:	Reardon, Peter, illustrator.
Dewey Number:	152.4

Printed in Australia by Minuteman Press Prahran 60086
Cover and interior design and illustrations by Peter Reardon, Pipeline Design (pipelinedesign.com.au)
Book production by Michael Hanrahan Publishing

This book does not constitute medical advice. If you are having health issues related to your grief it is important to get professional medical help.

For more information on Liz Crowe please go to LizCrowe.org or follow her on Twitter @LizCrowe2